VOLUME EATING DIET COOKBOOK FOR BEGINNERS

The Everything Guide to Volume Eating for Weight loss, Improved Digestion, Balanced Blood Sugar Level with Delicious Volumetrics Diet Recipes

Marian Elbert, RDN

work, encompassing digital renditions and forthcoming revisions.

TABLE OF CONTENTS

PART I: THE VOLUME EATING DIET

Consuming foods that are high in volume but low in calories is the main tenet of the volume eating diet. The basic premise is that people may control their calorie intake by eating more of some foods while consuming less of others. Volume eating promotes nutrient-dense, low-calorie meals that can help people feel full without going over their daily calorie restrictions, as opposed to restrictive diets that stress portion control and deprivation.

Consuming nutrient, water, and fiber-rich foods is an important part of the volume eating approach. Fruits, veggies, and whole grains are great sources of vitamins and minerals and help you feel full for longer. Many of these things have a high water content, which makes them bulkier and more filling without adding many to conventional dieting methods that stress calorie restriction and restriction of food intake, volume eating promotes the consumption of certain food groups that enable individuals to consume larger servings while still controlling their calorie consumption. For volume dieters, the most important thing is to eat meals with a low energy density, or few calories per gram.

Foods high in water and fiber are fundamental to the idea of volume eating. Particularly with volume eating, fruits and vegetables are preferred since they provide a lot of bulk without a lot of calories. People may find it easier to stick to a calorie-controlled eating plan if they include these items in their diet, as they make them feel fuller for longer.

Part of eating a lot of fruits and vegetables is making sure you consume nutrient-dense, natural meals with little processing. Some foods that can help you feel full without making you eat too many calories are whole grains, lean meats, and legumes. Promoting a balanced and healthy diet is the overarching objective, and this strategy is in line with it.

Meal planning with the goal of maximizing fullness is another facet of volume eating. Salads and broth-based soups are good examples of low-calorie, high-volume appetizers that can help control hunger and cut back on calories later in the meal. In this way, people may control their calorie consumption without sacrificing quantities of healthy food.

In general, concentrating on the quality and attributes of meals rather than simply restricting amount makes volume eating a more flexible and sustainable approach to healthy eating. Achieving health and weight management objectives without sacrificing savory, satisfying meals is possible when people focus on items that make them feel full without adding extra calories.

History of Volume Eating

Volume eating is based on a number of long-standing nutritional theories and dietary practices. Although *Volume Eating* was not used as a name until very recently, the concepts have been around in various forms in the field of nutrition and dietetics for quite some time.

The traditional diet's focus on whole, unadulterated foods is one historical precedent to volume eating. The concepts of volume eating were already present in societies that placed a premium on plant-based diets and whole grains. The dietary benefits of these foods, which were high in water and fiber, were known to these cultures, and they helped people feel full on less calories while still being healthy.

Research on the health advantages of whole foods contributed to a rising understanding of the need of dietary fiber in the middle of the twentieth century. The importance of fiber-rich meals in inducing fullness and sustaining digestive health started to get more attention from nutritionists and other health professionals. This period established the framework for the concept that, because of their makeup, some foods might be eaten in greater amounts without a commensurate increase in calories.

Thanks to the proliferation of health-related material online and the proliferation of social media, the idea of

consumption of legumes, whole grains, and certain fruits and vegetables, all of which are good providers of dietary fiber.

People that eat a lot of food also like to eat foods that are rich in nutrients, so their meals are usually not too heavy but yet include all the vitamins and minerals their bodies need. To promote health in all areas, this principle advocates eating a wide range of whole, minimally processed foods. Essential components of this part of volume eating include lean proteins, healthy fats, and a balanced intake of macronutrients.

Starting meals with low-calorie, high-volume components is another pillar of meal structure. Some people find that eating lighter appetizers like salads or broths before a major dinner helps them control their portion sizes. People may control their calorie consumption while enjoying larger servings overall using this method.

Essential principles of volume eating also include moderation and flexibility. This method promotes a reasonable and balanced perspective on eating rather than setting tight limitations. Volume eaters may maintain their eating habits for the long run by maintaining a healthy connection with food and allowing for occasional treats.

All things considered, the principles of volume eating include selecting low-calorie foods, eating foods that are rich in fiber and nutrients, planning meals so that you feel full after eating them, and being flexible and moderate with your food choices. Following these guidelines can help people achieve their health and wellness objectives while also providing a sustainable and enjoyable eating plan.

Volume Eating in Supporting Weight Management

Volume eating is a great tool for weight management since it provides a realistic and long-term strategy for regulating caloric intake. Choosing meals with a low calorie density is one of the main ways volume eating helps with weight management. In order to stay under their calorie restrictions, people should eat enough of water- and fiber-rich fruits, vegetables, and whole grains. In addition to making you feel fuller for longer, this aids in cutting calories, which is essential for losing weight.

Another important part of volume eating that helps with weight management is the emphasis on meals that are high in fiber. In addition to making you feel fuller for longer, the fiber in foods like legumes and whole grains slows your digestion, which means your body releases energy more gradually. This can aid in stabilizing blood sugar levels, which in turn reduces the risk of overeating and encourages a more regulated approach to calorie consumption by avoiding abrupt spikes and falls.

The consumption of nutrient-dense meals is promoted by volume eating, which further aids in weight management. Though they are low in calories, these meals are rich in many other nutrients that the body needs. In this way, people may be sure they are getting enough calories and other nutrients to maintain good health. By encouraging a healthy and well-rounded diet, this low-calorie density food item also helps with long-term weight management.

its best, it is crucial to strike a balance among these macronutrients.

Maintaining a healthy caloric balance is also important for people who are trying to control their weight. Although it is crucial to prioritize meals that are rich in nutrients, it is as necessary to watch the total number of calories consumed. Weight growth occurs when caloric intake exceeds energy expenditure, while weight decrease occurs when caloric intake is consistently lower than energy expenditure. People can fulfill their nutritional requirements and keep a healthy weight by finding a balance between the number of calories and the density of the nutrients.

Being conscious of portion sizes and making smart food choices are also important for maintaining a balance between nutrients and calories. For a well-rounded diet, it's best to eat a wide range of fruits, vegetables, lean meats, complete grains, and healthy fats. A well-balanced diet may be enhanced by opting for foods with little processing and preparing meals at home, where one has more control over the quality of the ingredients and the amount consumed.

Overall health and wellness are promoted by the interplay between calories and nutrients. Finding that sweet spot between over-and under-consumption of calories and essential nutrients is key to optimal health. An approach to nutrition that is both sustainable and health-conscious may be achieved by eating nutrient-dense meals while paying attention to the balance of macronutrients and controlling portions.

PART III: IMPACT OF HIGH-VOLUME FOODS

When it comes to encouraging fullness, controlling weight, and bolstering a healthy lifestyle, high-volume meals have a significant influence on eating habits and general health. When it comes to feeling full and satisfied without adding many calories to your diet, high-volume meals are essential. These foods are known for their low calorie density and high water and fiber content. For those trying to control their weight or make healthier food choices, this effect is especially helpful.

Increasing fullness is a noticeable side effect of eating more items with a high caloric content. Fruits and vegetables, which are rich in water, help you feel full for longer, which means you're less likely to overeat and more likely to limit your portion sizes. A more pleasurable and long-term strategy for controlling caloric intake is made possible by this enhanced fullness, which can be especially useful for people trying to reach or keep a healthy weight.

In terms of nutritional quality as a whole, high-volume meals are also beneficial. Fruits, vegetables, and whole grains are abundant in many of these items, and they are great sources of antioxidants, minerals, and vitamins. Individuals may help themselves achieve their weight loss goals and maintain optimal health by selecting nutrient-dense foods.

The total makeup of the diet might also be affected by the addition of meals with a large volume. Many people cut back on processed foods and energy-dense fruits and vegetables when they make the switch to a diet higher digestive system. In addition to aiding in the regulation of blood sugar levels, fiber promotes a healthy gut microbiota and controls bowel motions.

Carbohydrates, the body's principal energy source, are also contributed by meals that are high in volume. These foods may have less calories per serving, but the sugars, carbs, and fiber they provide are vital for proper carbohydrate metabolism. To maintain steady blood sugar levels and a steady stream of energy, load up on nutritious foods like sweet potatoes, quinoa, and oats, which are complex carbs.

Lean protein sources, like chicken, fish, lentils, and tofu, are abundant in high-volume diets and are an important source of protein, another macronutrient. Not only can these protein-rich foods help you feel full for longer, but they also aid in muscle repair and maintenance. People who are trying to control their weight or gain muscle may find that diets that are high in protein and volume are the most helpful.

Even while meals with a lot of volume don't usually have a lot of fat in them, they might include a little healthy fat like the kind you'd find in almonds, avocados, or olive oil. Incorporating these fats into the macronutrient profile helps with hormone synthesis and nutrition absorption, among other things.

All things considered, high-volume meals are a great source of many different macronutrients, such as fiber, carbs, proteins, and healthy fats. A well-rounded diet would be incomplete without these nutrient-dense alternatives, which contribute to general health, help with weight control, and make you feel full for longer.

best to eat plenty of water-rich meals like fruits and vegetables and drink enough water every day.

Proper heart and brain function depend on adequate intake of omega-3 and omega-6 fatty acids. Dietary supplies of these important fatty acids may be found in foods including walnuts, chia seeds, fatty fish, and flaxseeds. Maintaining healthy inflammation levels and cardiovascular function requires a balance between the two kinds of fatty acids.

A balanced diet includes a variety of nutrients, including water, vital fatty acids, vitamins, minerals, and macronutrients. If you want to keep your body's complex processes running smoothly, you need to eat a wide variety of foods. This includes fruits, vegetables, whole grains, lean meats, and healthy fats.

PART IV: LESS CALORIES MORE VOLUME RECIPES

BREAKFAST RECIPES FOR VOLUME EATING

Slow cooker vegetable curry

Ingredients

400ml can light coconut milk

3 tbsp mild curry paste

2 tsp vegetable bouillon powder

1 red chilli, deseeded and sliced

1 tbsp finely chopped ginger

3 garlic cloves, sliced

200g butternut squash (peeled weight), cut into chunks

1 red pepper, deseeded and sliced

1 small aubergine (about 250g), halved and thickly sliced

15g coriander, chopped

160g frozen peas, defrosted

1 lime, juiced, to taste

wholemeal flatbread, to serve

Method

STEP 1

Put the coconut milk, curry paste, bouillon powder, chilli, ginger, garlic, butternut squash, pepper and aubergine into the slow cooker pot and stir well. Cover with the lid and chill overnight.

STEP 2

Cook on low for 6 hrs until the vegetables are really tender, then stir in the coriander and defrosted peas. The heat of the curry should be enough to warm them through. Taste and add a good squeeze of lime juice, if you fancy extra zing. Serve with a wholemeal flatbread.

Green chowder with prawns

Ingredients

1 tbsp olive oil

1 onion, finely chopped

1 celery stick, finely chopped

1 garlic clove

300g petit pois

200g pack sliced kale

2 potatoes, finely chopped

1 low-salt chicken stock cube (we used Kallo)

100g cooked North Atlantic prawns

Method

STEP 1

Heat the oil in a saucepan over a medium heat. Add the onion and celery and cook for 5-6 mins until softened but not coloured. Add the garlic and cook for a further min. Stir in the petit pois, kale and potatoes, then add the stock cube and 750ml water. Bring to the boil and simmer for 10-12 mins until the potatoes are soft.

STEP 2

Tip ¾ of the mixture into a food processor and whizz until smooth. Add a little more water or stock if it's too thick. Pour the mixture back into the pan and add half the prawns.

STEP 3

Divide between four bowls and spoon the remaining prawns on top. Can be frozen for up to a month. Add the prawns once defrosted.

Healthy pesto eggs on toast

Ingredients

2-4 thin slices rye sourdough (about 70g total, depending on the size of the loaf)

2 eggs

170g tomatoes on-the-vine

160g baby spinach

pinch of chilli flakes (optional)

For the pesto

1 garlic clove

10g basil

1 tbsp pine nuts

1 tbsp rapeseed oil

1 tbsp finely grated parmesan or vegetarian alternative

Method

STEP 1

To make the pesto, peel the garlic clove and put in a small food processor along with the basil, pine nuts, oil and 2 tbsp water. Blitz until smooth, then stir in the cheese. Or, blitz using a hand blender.

STEP 2

Toast the bread and divide between two plates. Cook the pesto in a frying pan over a medium heat for 30 seconds, stirring. Crack the eggs into one side of the pan, put the tomatoes in the other, and fry in the pesto until the eggs are cooked to your liking.

STEP 3

Lift out the eggs and put each one on a slice of toast. Add the spinach to the pan with the tomatoes, turn the heat up to high and cook until wilted, about 2-3 mins. The tomatoes should be soft. Spoon the veg onto the other toast slice and sprinkle with the chilli flakes, if you like

Somerset stew with cheddar & parsley mash

Ingredients

1 tbsp oil

1 onion, finely chopped

1 garlic clove, finely chopped

1 large carrot, finely chopped

1 leek, chopped

1 tbsp tomato purée

400g can chopped tomato

200g can butter bean, drained

400g can flageolet bean, rinsed and drained

200ml dry cider, or additional stock

250ml vegetable stock

few sprigs thyme, leaves only

cheddar & parsley mash (see tip below)

Make it non-veggie

2 sausages

1 tsp olive oil per portion

a few, or one, of the following to serve: crumbled feta cheese (or a dairy-free alternative), chopped spring onions, sliced radishes, avocado chunks, soured cream

Method

STEP 1

In a large pot, heat the olive oil and fry the garlic and onions for 5 mins until almost softened. Add the pimenton and cumin, cook for a few mins, then add the vinegar, sugar, tomatoes and some seasoning. Cook for 10 mins.

STEP 2

Pour in the beans and cook for another 10 mins. Serve with rice and the accompaniments of your choice in small bowls

Aubergine & chickpea stew

Ingredients

200g dried chickpeas, soaked for 6-8 hours

2 tbsp extra virgin olive oil, plus extra to serve (optional)

2 onions, finely sliced

6 garlic cloves, crushed

1 tbsp baharat

1 tsp ground cinnamon

1 small bunch of flat-leaf parsley, stalks finely chopped, leaves roughly chopped, to serve

3 medium aubergines, sliced into 2cm rounds

2 x 400g cans chopped tomatoes

1 lemon, juiced

50g pine nuts, toasted, to serve

pitta breads or flatbreads, to serve (optional)

Method

STEP 1

Drain the chickpeas and bring to the boil in a pan of salted water. Cook for 10 mins, then drain.

STEP 2

Heat the oil in a frying pan over a medium heat and fry the onions for 10 mins, or until beginning to soften. Stir in the garlic, baharat and cinnamon and cook for 1 min. Tip the onion mixture into a slow cooker and add the chickpeas, parsley stalks, aubergines, tomatoes and a can of water. Season. Cover and cook on high for 2 hrs, then turn the heat to low and cook for 6-8 hrs more until the mixture has reduced slightly and the chickpeas and aubergines are really tender.

STEP 3

Stir in the lemon juice, then scatter over the pine nuts and parsley leaves. Drizzle over some extra olive oil and serve with pitta breads or flatbreads, if you like

Healthy Halloween stuffed peppers

Ingredients

4 small peppers (a mix of orange, red and yellow looks nice)

25g pine nuts

1 tbsp olive or rapeseed oil

1 red onion, chopped

2 fat garlic cloves, crushed

1 small aubergine, chopped into small pieces

200g pouch mixed grains (we used bulghur wheat and quinoa)

2 tbsp sundried tomato paste

zest of 1 lemon

bunch basil, chopped

Method

STEP 1

Cut the tops off the peppers (keeping the tops to one side) and remove the seeds and any white flesh from inside. Use a small sharp knife to carve spooky Halloween faces into the sides. Chop any offcuts into small pieces and set aside.

STEP 2

Toast the pine nuts in a dry pan for a few mins until golden, and set aside. Heat the oil in the pan, and heat the oven to 200C/180C fan/gas 6. Cook the onion in the oil for 8-10 mins until softened. Stir in the garlic, pepper offcuts and aubergine and cook for another 10 mins, until the veggies are soft. Add a splash of water if the pan looks dry. Season.

STEP 3

Squeeze the pouch of grains to break them up, then tip into the pan with the tomato paste. Stir for a minute or two to warm through, then remove from the heat and add the lemon zest, basil and pine nuts.

STEP 4

Fill each pepper with the grain mixture. Replace the lids, using cocktail sticks to secure them in place, and put the peppers in a deep roasting tin with the carved faces facing upwards. Cover with foil and bake for 35 mins, uncovered for the final 10. The peppers should be soft and the filling piping hot

Healthy pesto eggs on toast

Ingredients

2-4 thin slices rye sourdough (about 70g total, depending on the size of the loaf)

2 eggs

170g tomatoes on-the-vine

160g baby spinach

pinch of chilli flakes (optional)

For the pesto

1 garlic clove

10g basil

1 tbsp pine nuts

50g cherry tomatoes, halved

15g feta , crumbled

Method

STEP 1

Bring a large pan of water to the boil. Heat the oil in a frying pan over a medium heat and add the kale, garlic and chilli flakes. Cook, stirring occasionally, for 4 mins until the kale begins to crisp and wilt to half its size. Set aside.

STEP 2

Adjust the heat so the water is at a rolling boil, then poach your eggs for 2 mins. Meanwhile, toast the bread.

STEP 3

Remove the poached eggs with a slotted spoon and top each piece of toast with half the kale, an egg, the cherry tomatoes and feta.

Porridge with blueberry compote

Ingredients

6 tbsp porridge oats

just under ½ x 200ml tub 0% fat Greek-style yogurt

½ x 350g pack frozen blueberries

1 tsp honey (optional)

Method

STEP 1

Put the oats in a non-stick pan with 400ml water and cook over the heat, stirring occasionally for about 2 minutes until thickened. Remove from the heat and add a third of the yogurt.

STEP 2

Meanwhile, tip the blueberries into a pan with 1 tbsp water and the honey if using and gently poach until the blueberries have thawed and they are tender, but still holding their shape.

STEP 3

Spoon the porridge into bowls, top with the remaining yogurt and spoon over the blueberries.

Eggy spelt bread with orange cheese & raspberries

Ingredients

2 medium eggs

2 tbsp orange juice

2 slices spelt bread, halved

50g low-fat cottage cheese

1 tsp orange zest

1 tsp rapeseed oil

50g raspberries

clear honey, to serve (optional)

Method

STEP 1

Beat the eggs and orange juice in a bowl wide enough to fit the bread in it. Soak the bread in the eggs and juice for 2 mins or so, turning halfway through.

STEP 2

Meanwhile, in a small bowl, mix together the cheese and orange zest. Put the rapeseed oil in a non-stick

1 tsp oil

80g chestnut mushrooms, sliced

50g ham, diced

80g bag spinach

4 medium eggs, beaten

1 tbsp grated cheddar

Method

STEP 1

Heat the grill to its highest setting. Heat the oil in an ovenproof frying pan over a medium-high heat. Tip in the mushrooms and fry for 2 mins until mostly softened. Stir in the ham and spinach, and cook for 1 min more until the spinach has wilted. Season well with black pepper and a pinch of salt.

STEP 2

Reduce the heat and pour over the eggs. Cook undisturbed for 3 mins until the eggs are mostly set. Sprinkle over the cheese and put under the grill for 2 mins. Serve hot or cold.

Veggie breakfast bakes

Ingredients

4 large field mushrooms

8 tomatoes, halved

1 garlic clove, thinly sliced

2 tsp olive oil

200g bag spinach

4 eggs

Method

STEP 1

Heat oven to 200C/180C fan/gas 6. Put the mushrooms and tomatoes into 4 ovenproof dishes. Divide garlic between the dishes, drizzle over the oil and some seasoning, then bake for 10 mins.

STEP 2

Meanwhile, put the spinach into a large colander, then pour over a kettle of boiling water to wilt it. Squeeze out any excess water, then add the spinach to the dishes. Make a little gap between the vegetables and crack an egg into each dish. Return to the oven and cook for a further 8-10 mins or until the egg is cooked to your liking.

Spiced fruit loaf

Ingredients

For the dough

450g strong white flour, plus extra for dusting

2 x 7g sachets easy-blend yeast

50g caster sugar

150ml warm milk

1 egg, beaten

50g unsalted butter, melted, plus extra for greasing

oil, for greasing

For the spices

1½ tsp ground cinnamon

1 tsp ground ginger

For the dried fruit

50g dried apricot, chopped

Egg Niçoise salad

Ingredients

For the dressing

2 tbsp rapeseed oil

juice 1 lemon

1 tsp balsamic vinegar

1 garlic clove, grated

⅓ small pack basil, leaves chopped

3 pitted black Kalamata olive, rinsed and chopped

For the salad

2 eggs

250g new potatoes, thickly sliced

200g fine green beans

½ red onion, very finely chopped

14 cherry tomatoes, halved

6 romaine lettuces leaves, torn into bite-sized pieces

6 pitted black Kalamata olive, rinsed and halved

Method

STEP 1

Mix the dressing **Ingredients** together in a small bowl with 1 tbsp water.

STEP 2

Meanwhile boil the potatoes for 7 mins, add the beans and boil 5 mins more or until both are just tender, then drain. Boil 2 eggs for 8 minutes then shell and halve.

STEP 3

Toss the beans, potatoes and remaining salad ingredients, except the eggs, together in a large bowl with half the dressing. Arrange the eggs on top and drizzle over the remaining dressing

Griddled salad jar

Ingredients

1 aubergine, sliced

1 courgette, sliced

1 tbsp olive oil

2 tomatoes, roughly chopped

200g feta, roughly crumbled

240g can chickpeas

100g Kalamata olives

50g sundried tomatoes

¼ cucumber, deseeded and roughly chopped

1 yellow pepper, deseeded and sliced

small bunch mint, leaves only

small bunch dill, chopped

For the pickled onion dressing

1 red onion, sliced

½ tsp coriander seeds

50ml white wine vinegar

juice 1 lemon

100ml extra virgin olive oil

Method

STEP 1

To make the dressing, put the onion in a medium-sized pan and heat gently with the coriander seeds, vinegar and 50ml water for 15 mins or until the onion is bright pink and soft. Put the pan to one side to cool.

STEP 2

Heat a griddle pan until smoking hot, then brush the aubergines and courgette slices with a little olive oil. Griddle for 3-4 mins each side until char lines appear. Transfer to a plate, season well and leave to cool.

STEP 3

Whisk the lemon juice then the olive oil into the pan with the cooled onion. Season and tip into the jar. To build your salad, layer in the tomatoes followed by the feta, chickpeas and olives. Push everything down a little, then add the sundried tomatoes and some of their oil. Add your griddled vegetables, followed by the cucumber, pepper and herbs. Put on the lid and leave in the fridge or a cool box until you're ready to eat.

STEP 4

To serve, tip out onto a serving platter so the dressing is drizzled over the top of everything last

Vegan leek & potato soup

Ingredients

1 tbsp rapeseed oil, plus a drizzle to serve (optional)

2 large garlic cloves, chopped

500g leeks, thinly sliced

500g potatoes, cut into cubes

500ml vegan vegetable stock, made with 1½ tsp bouillon powder

500ml unsweetened almond milk

chopped chives and bread, to serve

Method

STEP 1

Heat the oil in a large pan over a medium heat and fry the garlic and leeks, stirring, until the veg has started to soften. Add the potatoes and stock, then cover and simmer for 15 mins until the leeks and potatoes are soft.

STEP 2

Pour in the almond milk, then remove from the heat and blitz using a hand blender until almost smooth, with a slightly chunky texture. Or, if you prefer, blitz until completely smooth. Reheat over a low heat if needed, then ladle into bowls and scatter with chives, drizzle with a little oil and serve with bread, if you like. Can be frozen for up to three months

Tomato & black bean taco salad

Ingredients

1 lime, juiced

12g coriander, finely chopped

½ tsp ground cumin

1 jalapeño pepper (deseeded if you prefer less heat), finely chopped

2 tbsp rapeseed oil

400g can black beans, drained and rinsed

200g cherry tomatoes, halved

1 romaine lettuce, chopped

198g can sweetcorn, drained

1 red pepper, finely chopped

4 crunchy taco shells

25g pumpkin seeds

Method

STEP 1

Combine the lime juice, coriander, cumin, jalapeño and oil in a bowl. Season well.

STEP 2

Tip in the beans, tomatoes, lettuce, corn and red pepper. Toss to combine. Crumble in the taco shells and mix to coat everything in the dressing. Scatter over the pumpkin seeds and serve straightaway.

Ponzu tofu poke bowl

Ingredients

1 tbsp ponzu sauce

½ tbsp rice vinegar

5g ginger, peeled and grated

1 tsp sesame oil

300g silken tofu

100g edamame beans

250g pouch cooked quinoa

100g radishes, sliced

2 carrots, peeled into ribbons

2 spring onions, finely sliced

2 small seaweed thins, crumbled

1 tsp sesame seeds

Method

STEP 1

Combine the ponzu, vinegar, ginger and sesame oil in a bowl. Pat the tofu dry using kitchen paper and tear into chunks, then gently toss in the ponzu mixture.

STEP 2

Pour some boiling water over the edamame and set aside for 2 mins before draining thoroughly and seasoning with salt.

STEP 3

Divide the quinoa between bowls and top with the edamame, radishes and carrots. Spoon over the tofu and drizzle over the remaining dressing before scattering over the spring onions, seaweed and sesame seeds

Red pepper & potato omelette

Ingredients

3 tbsp olive oil

2 small red peppers, deseeded, halved and finely sliced

2 medium potatoes, finely sliced

8 eggs

Method

STEP 1

Heat 2 tbsp oil in a medium non-stick frying pan over a medium-low heat and cook the peppers and potatoes for 10 mins until softened – if the pan has a lid, cover it to speed things up. Meanwhile, beat the eggs in a large bowl with some seasoning. When the potatoes and peppers are cooked, tip them into the eggs and stir to combine – the heat from the veg will start to cook the eggs.

STEP 2

Heat the grill to high. Heat the rest of the oil in the pan over a medium heat, tip in the egg and veg mixture, and cook, stirring occasionally with a spatula and drawing the edges into the middle, until nearly set, about 5-6 mins. Slide the pan under the grill for a few minutes to just set the top, then slide the omelette onto a plate. Flip it back into the pan and finish cooking the omelette on the underside for another few minutes, being careful not to burn it.

STEP 3

Turn the omelette out onto a board and leave to cool. Serve in wedges in a lunchbox, or slice and stuff into a baguette or crusty roll

Vegan chickpea curry jacket potatoes

Ingredients

4 sweet potatoes

1 tbsp coconut oil

1 ½ tsp cumin seeds

1 large onion, diced

2 garlic cloves, crushed

thumb-sized piece ginger, finely grated

1 green chilli, finely chopped

1 tsp garam masala

1 tsp ground coriander

½ tsp turmeric

2 tbsp tikka masala paste

2 x 400g can chopped tomatoes

2 x 400g can chickpeas, drained

lemon wedges and coriander leaves, to serve

Method

STEP 1

Heat oven to 200C/180C fan/gas 6. Prick the sweet potatoes all over with a fork, then put on a baking tray and roast in the oven for 45 mins or until tender when pierced with a knife.

STEP 2

Meanwhile, melt the coconut oil in a large saucepan over medium heat. Add the cumin seeds and fry for 1 min until fragrant, then add the onion and fry for 7-10 mins until softened.

STEP 3

Put the garlic, ginger and green chilli into the pan, and cook for 2-3 mins. Add the spices and tikka masala paste and cook for a further 2 mins until fragrant, then tip in the tomatoes. Bring to a simmer, then tip in the chickpeas and cook for a further 20 mins until thickened. Season.

STEP 4

Put the roasted sweet potatoes on four plates and cut open lengthways. Spoon over the chickpea curry and squeeze over the lemon wedges. Season, then scatter with coriander before serving.

Healthy carrot soup

Ingredients

3 large carrots

1 tbsp grated ginger

1 tsp turmeric

a pinch of cayenne pepper, plus extra to serve

20g wholemeal bread

1 tbsp soured cream, plus extra to serve

200ml vegetable stock

Method

STEP 1

Peel and chop the carrots and put in a blender with the ginger, turmeric, cayenne pepper, wholemeal bread, soured cream and vegetable stock. Blitz until smooth. Heat until piping hot. Swirl through some extra soured cream, or a sprinkling of cayenne, if you like.

Halloumi, carrot & orange salad

Ingredients

2 large oranges

1½ tbsp wholegrain mustard

1½ tsp honey

1 tbsp white wine vinegar

3 tbsp rapeseed or olive oil, plus extra for frying

2 large carrots, peeled

225g block halloumi, sliced

100g bag watercress or baby spinach

Method

STEP 1

Cut the peel and pith away from the oranges. Use a small serrated knife to segment the orange, catching any juices in a bowl, then squeeze any excess juice from the off-cut pith into the bowl as well. Add the mustard, honey, vinegar, oil and some seasoning to the bowl and mix well.

STEP 2

Using a vegetable peeler, peel carrot ribbons into the dressing bowl and toss gently. Heat a drizzle of oil in a frying pan and cook the halloumi for a few mins until golden on both sides. Toss the watercress through the dressed carrots. Arrange the watercress mixture on plates and top with the halloumi and oranges

Orzo & chickpea soup

Ingredients

2 tbsp olive oil

1 onion, chopped

2 carrots, chopped

2 celery sticks, chopped

2 tbsp tomato purée

3 garlic cloves, chopped

3 rosemary or thyme sprigs

1 litre vegetable stock

400g can chopped tomatoes

400g can chickpeas

parmesan rind or vegetarian alternative (optional)

150g orzo

extra virgin olive oil, to serve

Method

STEP 1

Heat the olive oil in a deep pan over a medium-high heat and cook the onion, carrots and celery, including any leaves for 15 mins until softened. Stir in the tomato purée, garlic cloves and rosemary or thyme sprigs. Cook for a few minutes until the purée is caramelised. Pour in the stock, chopped tomatoes, chickpeas (and the liquid from the can) and parmesan rind, if you have one. Simmer 15 mins.

STEP 2

Pour boiling water over the orzo in a heatproof bowl and set aside for 15 mins. Drain the orzo, add to the pan and cook for 5-8 mins until the orzo is tender. Fish out and discard the rosemary stalks and cheese rind, then season well. Drizzle over extra virgin olive oil and grated cheese to serve.

Smoky chickpea salad

Ingredients

1 tbsp sunflower oil

2 x 400g can chickpeas, drained and rinsed

200g carrots, peeled into ribbons or grated

200g spinach

1 small head of broccoli, roughly chopped

For the dressing

2 tsp smoked paprika

2 tsp garlic granules

2 tsp dried mixed herbs

4 tsp maple syrup

2 tbsp low-sodium soy sauce

4 tsp rice vinegar

2 tsp sesame oil

Method

STEP 1

Heat the oil in a large pan over a medium heat. Tip in the chickpeas and fry gently for 3-4 mins until sizzling and slightly crispy.

STEP 2

Whisk together the dressing **Ingredients** in a bowl, then pour over the chickpeas along with 4 tbsp water and bring to a boil. Cook for 1-2 mins until reduced slightly, remove from the heat, season well and set aside.

STEP 3

Toss the carrots, spinach and raw broccoli together and divide between plates. Scatter over the chickpeas and a spoonful of the pan juices to dress.

Sweet potato toasts with curried chickpeas

Ingredients

3 large sweet potatoes (about 350g), trimmed and thinly sliced lengthways into 12

rapeseed oil, for brushing (about 1 tsp)

For the chickpeas

2 tbsp rapeseed oil

150g celery, finely chopped

3 garlic cloves, finely grated

2 tbsp mild curry powder

1 tsp cumin seeds

400g can chopped tomatoes

2 tbsp tomato purée

1½ tsp vegetable bouillon powder

2 x 400g cans chickpeas, drained

365g frozen spinach

⅓ x 30g pack of coriander, chopped

Method

STEP 1

Heat the oven to 200C/180C fan/gas 6. Brush the sweet potato slices with a little oil, arrange in a single layer on a baking tray, then bake for 20-25 mins. Check towards the end to make sure they are not catching – move around if the slices near the edges of the tray are browning faster than the ones in the middle.

STEP 2

For the chickpeas, heat the oil in a large pan over a medium heat and fry the celery for 5 mins, stirring frequently. Add the garlic, curry powder and cumin seeds, stir briefly, then tip in the tomatoes, tomato purée and bouillon. Stir in the chickpeas and frozen spinach, then cover and simmer for 15 mins. Stir in the coriander.

STEP 3

Divide half the chickpeas between six pieces of the sweet potato toast, and serve three toasts per person. Cool and chill the rest to eat another day. To serve, reheat the chickpeas in a pan over a low heat with a splash of water until piping hot. Briefly heat the sweet potato slices in a dry frying pan over a low heat, watching carefully so they don't burn. Will keep chilled for three days.

BLT pasta salad

Ingredients

25g pasta bows

2 cooked crispy bacon rashers, broken into pieces

15g spinach, chopped

6 cherry tomatoes, halved

½ tbsp crème fraîche

¼ tsp wholegrain mustard

Method

STEP 1

The night before school, cook the pasta following pack instructions and run under cold water to cool quickly. Mix in the bacon, spinach, tomatoes, crème fraîche and mustard, and season with a little salt. Spoon into an airtight container and keep overnight in the fridge.

Teriyaki tofu

Ingredients

1 tbsp olive oil

400g firm tofu, cut into bite-sized cubes

1 large head of broccoli, cut into florets, stalks peeled and thinly sliced

1 bunch of spring onions, separated into white and green parts and thinly sliced

8-10 tbsp teriyaki sauce

cooked rice or noodles, to serve

Method

STEP 1

Heat the oil in a pan over a medium heat and fry the tofu for about 8 mins until crisp and golden. Remove from the pan and set aside.

STEP 2

In the same pan, add the broccoli florets and white parts of the spring onions and cook for around 4 mins until tender, but not completely cooked through. Stir in the teriyaki sauce and season well.

STEP 3

Add the cooked tofu back to the pan with the broccoli and stir well to coat. Cook for an additional 1-2 mins for the flavours to meld together. Sprinkle over the reserved green parts of the spring onions, remove from the heat and serve with cooked rice or noodles.

DINNER RECIPES FOR VOLUME EATING

Egg-fried noodles with beansprouts

Ingredients

2 dried wholemeal noodle nests (about 100g)

2 limes, juiced

1 tsp tamari

2 garlic cloves, 1 finely grated, 1 chopped

1 red chilli, deseeded and finely sliced

1 tbsp sesame or rapeseed oil

2 red onions, (200g), halved and thinly sliced

15g ginger, peeled and cut into fine shreds

1 small red pepper, deseeded and cut into strips

1 tbsp medium curry powder

200g ready-to-eat beansprouts, rinsed and drained

1 tbsp tahini

3 eggs, beaten

15g coriander, chopped

Method

STEP 1

Cook the noodles following pack instructions. Combine the lime juice, tamari, grated garlic and chilli in a small bowl. Set aside.

STEP 2

Heat the oil in a non-stick wok or large, wide pan over a high heat and stir-fry the onions, ginger and pepper for 5 mins until softened (add the chopped garlic for the last minute). Stir in the curry powder and cook for a minute more. Add the beansprouts and continue cooking until the beansprouts start to soften and are piping hot. Mix in the tahini.

STEP 3

Push the veg to the side of the wok and pour in the egg – you may need a drop more oil. Stir-fry the eggs so they are mostly set, then stir the veg into the egg and add the noodles and coriander, then toss to combine. Pile into bowls and serve with the sauce on the side.

Slow-cooker chickpea stew

Ingredients

1 tbsp vegetable or sunflower oil

1 red onion, sliced

2 garlic cloves, crushed or finely grated

1 butternut squash (around 600g), deseeded and cut into bite-size chunks

½ tsp ground ginger

1 tsp ground cumin

1 tsp smoked paprika

1 tsp ground coriander

1 tsp ground turmeric

½ tsp ground cinnamon

400g can chickpeas

400g can chopped tomatoes

2 tbsp tomato purée

500ml vegetable stock

cooked couscous and a handful of coriander, chopped, to serve

Method

STEP 1

Heat the oil in a large frying pan or saucepan over a medium-low heat and fry the onion for 10-12 mins until softened and beginning to turn golden. Stir in the garlic and cook for 1 min, then add the squash and cook for a few minutes more to soften slightly. Scatter in the spices, stir to combine, and cook for 2 mins until fragrant.

STEP 2

Tip everything in the pan into the slow cooker along with the chickpeas and their liquid, the tomatoes, tomato purée and the stock. Mix well, then cook on high for 5 hrs or low for 7 hrs. Serve alongside couscous, with the coriander sprinkled over.

Sardine tomato pasta with gremolata

Ingredients

75g wholemeal spaghetti

1/2 x 120g can sardines in oil

½ tbsp capers, drained

2 garlic cloves, crushed

2 tomatoes, roughly chopped

30g rocket

½ lemon, zested

small handful of parsley, finely chopped

Method

STEP 1

Cook the pasta following pack instructions in a large pan of boiling salted water. Heat 1 tbsp oil from the can of sardines in a non-stick frying pan over a medium heat and sizzle the capers and half the garlic for 1-2 mins until fragrant. Tip in the tomatoes and fry for 4-5 mins more until softened and bursting. Stir in the sardines and rocket, tossing a few times to break up the fish and wilt the leaves. Season.

STEP 2

For the gremolata, combine the lemon zest, parsley and remaining garlic in a small bowl, and season. Drain the pasta and top with the sardine sauce and gremolata.

Coconut & squash dhansak

Ingredients

1 tbsp vegetable oil

500g butternut squash (about 1 small squash), peeled and chopped into bite-sized chunks (or buy a pack of ready-prepared to save time), see tip, below left

100g frozen chopped onions

4 heaped tbsp mild curry paste (we used korma)

400g can chopped tomatoes

400g can light coconut milk

mini naan bread, to serve

400g can lentils, drained

200g bag baby spinach

150ml coconut yogurt (we used Rachel's Organic), plus extra to serve

Method

STEP 1

Heat the oil in a large pan. Put the squash in a bowl with a splash of water. Cover with cling film and microwave on High for 10 mins or until tender. Meanwhile, add the onions to the hot oil and cook for a few mins until soft. Add the curry paste, tomatoes and coconut milk, and simmer for 10 mins until thickened to a rich sauce.

STEP 2

Warm the naan breads in a low oven or in the toaster. Drain any liquid from the squash, then add to the sauce with the lentils, spinach and some seasoning. Simmer for a further 2-3 mins to wilt the spinach, then stir in the coconut yogurt. Serve with the warm naan and a dollop of extra yogurt.

Harissa fish with bulgur salad

Ingredients

100g bulgur wheat

½ small cucumber, deseeded and finely chopped

100g cherry tomatoes, quartered

25g pitted green olives

small handful of parsley, finely chopped

2tbsp rose harissa

2tsp honey

1 garlic clove, crushed

½ lemon, juiced

2tbsp olive oil

½ red onion, finely sliced

2 x 120g skinless, boneless white fish fillets, such as cod
or haddock

Method

STEP 1

Cook the bulgur following pack instructions, then rinse and drain well before tipping into a large bowl. Add the cucumber, tomatoes, olives and most of the parsley. Season well. Combine the harissa, honey, garlic, lemon juice, half the oil and 1 tbsp water in a bowl, then set aside.

STEP 2

Heat the remaining oil in a non-stick pan over a medium heat and cook the red onion for 4-5 mins until softened and lightly browned. Season the fish well, then add to the pan and cook for 3 mins before pouring in the harissa mixture. Turn the fish and cook for 2-4 mins more (depending on the thickness of the fish), basting the fish in the pan juices until cooked through – the flesh should be opaque.

STEP 3

Divide the bulgur salad between two plates, top with the fish and fried onions, then drizzle over any remaining pan juices and sprinkle over the remaining parsley to serve.

Courgette, chilli & mint with pearl couscous

Ingredients

100g pearl couscous

1 tbsp olive oil

400g courgettes, roughly chopped

½ red onion, sliced

1 red chilli (deseeded if you prefer less heat), finely chopped

2 garlic cloves, finely sliced

10g mint, leaves picked and finely chopped, plus a few whole to serve

½ lemon, juiced

1 tbsp honey

50g light Greek-style salad cheese

Method

STEP 1

Cook the couscous following pack instructions, then drain and set aside. Meanwhile, heat the oil in a frying pan over a medium-high heat. Tip in the courgettes and onion and fry, stirring occasionally, until browned and softened, about 8-10 mins. Stir in the chilli and garlic and cook for a further 2-3 mins until fragrant.

STEP 2

Remove from the heat and stir through the chopped mint, lemon juice, honey and seasoning. Divide the couscous between plates, top with the courgette mix, crumble over the cheese and scatter with the whole mint leaves to serve.

Ginger chicken udon noodles

Ingredients

1 tsp sunflower oil

3 boneless, skinless chicken thighs, diced

¼ white cabbage, finely sliced

25g ginger, peeled and finely grated

1 red chilli (deseeded if you like), finely chopped

1 tbsp low-salt soy sauce

2 tsp rice vinegar

2 tsp mirin

100g ready-to-eat beansprouts

3 spring onions, finely sliced

300g straight-to-wok udon noodles

small handful of coriander, finely chopped

1 tbsp pickled ginger (optional)

Method

STEP 1

Heat the oil in a large, deep frying pan over a medium-high heat and, once hot, stir-fry the chicken and cabbage for 5-7 mins until browned and almost cooked through. Add the ginger and chilli, and cook for a few minutes more until fragrant.

STEP 2

Add the remaining ingredients, except the coriander and pickled ginger, and fry until the chicken is cooked and the noodles are tender, about 1-2 mins more. Season, adding more soy, vinegar or mirin, if you like. Top with the coriander and pickled ginger, if using.

Gingery broccoli-fry with cashews

Ingredients

320g head of broccoli, stalks and florets separated

40g cashews, roughly chopped

1 tbsp sesame oil

15g ginger, finely sliced

1 small red onion, finely chopped

1 red pepper, deseeded and cut into thin strips

1 large carrot (160g), cut into thin strips

2 garlic cloves, thinly sliced

1 red chilli, deseeded and finely chopped, plus extra sliced, to serve

1 tbsp tamari

1 lime, juiced and zested

7g chopped coriander, plus extra to serve

2 eggs, beaten

Method

STEP 1

Blitz the broccoli stalks in a food processor until finely chopped. Add the florets and pulse again to achieve a rice-like texture.

STEP 2

Lightly toast the cashews in a wok or frying pan, then tip onto a plate and set aside. Heat the oil in a pan over a high heat and add the ginger, onion, pepper, carrot, garlic and chilli. Stir-fry for 2-3 mins until starting to brown, then put a lid on and cook for another 2 mins.

STEP 3

Add the broccoli and 3 tbsp water and stir-fry for 3 mins until all the veg is tender. Pour in the tamari, lime juice and zest and coriander, stir well, then pour in the eggs and stir-fry very briefly to just set. Serve with the cashews, extra coriander and extra sliced chilli scattered over, if you like.

Poached salmon with tarragon

Ingredients

1 lemon

200g half-fat crème fraîche

small pack tarragon, leaves only, chopped

1 garlic clove, crushed to a paste

400g green beans, trimmed and halved

4 salmon fillets

cooked baby new potatoes, to serve

Method

STEP 1

Zest the lemon and cut into wedges. Mix together the crème fraîche, tarragon, garlic, lemon zest and a squeeze of juice, season to taste and set aside.

STEP 2

Bring a large shallow pan of salted water to the bowl and cook the green beans for 3 mins until just done. Remove with a slotted spoon, drain and cool under cold running water before tossing with the crème fraîche mixture.

STEP 3

Bring the pan back to the boil, then turn the heat down to a very gentle simmer and slide in the salmon pieces. Poach for 8-10 mins or until cooked to your liking. Remove from the pan and put on kitchen paper before plating up. Serve with the green beans and baby new potatoes

Healthy tikka masala

Ingredients

1 large onion, chopped

4 large garlic cloves

thumb-sized piece of ginger

2 tbsp rapeseed oil

4 small skinless chicken breasts, cut into chunks

2 tbsp tikka spice powder

1 tsp cayenne pepper

400g can chopped tomatoes

40g ground almonds

200g spinach

3 tbsp fat-free natural yogurt

½ small bunch of coriander, chopped

brown basmati rice, to serve

Method

STEP 1

Put the onion, garlic and ginger in a food processor and whizz to a smooth paste.

STEP 2

Heat 1 tbsp of the oil in a flameproof casserole dish over a medium heat. Add the onion mixture and fry for 15 mins. Tip into a bowl and wipe out the pan.

STEP 3

Add the remaining oil and the chicken and fry for 5-7 mins, or until lightly brown. Stir in the tikka spice and cayenne and fry for a further minute. Tip the onion mixture back into the pan, along with the tomatoes and 1 can full of water. Bring to the boil, then reduce to a simmer and cook, uncovered, for 15 mins. Stir in the almonds and spinach and cook for a further 10 mins. Season, then stir though the yogurt and coriander. Serve with brown rice.

Fajita chicken one-pot

Ingredients

2 tsp olive oil

200g cooking chorizo, roughly chopped

6 boneless and skinless chicken thighs, roughly chopped

2 red onions, roughly chopped

2 Romano peppers, roughly chopped

1½ tbsp fajita seasoning

400g can pinto beans, drained and rinsed

350g new potatoes, halved, or quartered if large

300ml chicken stock, made with 1 stock cube

3 corn on the cobs, halved or quartered

100g soured cream, to serve

handful of parsley, chopped, to serve (optional)

Method

STEP 1

Heat the oil in a large, lidded, heavy-based saucepan over a medium heat and fry the chorizo for 4 mins to release the oils and brown it a little. Remove to a plate using a slotted spoon and set aside. Fry the chicken for 5-6 mins until browned but not cooked all the way through. You may need to do this in batches. Remove with the slotted spoon and set aside with the chorizo.

STEP 2

Add the onions and peppers to the pan and cook, stirring often for 6-8 mins until softened and starting to lightly brown. Use a wooden spoon to scrape up any caramelised bits on the bottom and mix them in. Stir in the fajita seasoning and cook for 30 seconds before returning the chorizo and chicken to the pan.

STEP 3

Season with salt and freshly ground black pepper and give everything a good stir. Tip in the pinto beans and potatoes, stir to coat well, then pour in the stock, topping up with water if it doesn't cover the chicken and veg. Bring to a simmer, reduce the heat a little and put the lid on. Simmer gently for 10 mins. Give everything a stir, then sit the corn on the cobs on top.

STEP 4

Return the lid to the pan and cook for a further 15 mins. Serve in large bowls, each topped with a spoonful of soured cream and a scattering of chopped parsley, if you like.

Sweet potato wedges with mole sauce

Ingredients

450g courgettes, cut into thick wedges

300g small sweet potatoes, cut into thick wedges

2½ tsp olive oil

1 red onion, halved and thinly sliced

½ lime, juiced

1 onion, finely chopped

1 tbsp chopped thyme

400g can chopped tomatoes

½ tsp vegetable bouillon powder

3 tbsp crunchy peanut butter

15g raisins, finely chopped

1 tsp smoked paprika

¼ tsp habanero chilli flakes (optional)

1 cinnamon stick

400g can black beans

2 tsp ground cumin

3 garlic cloves, finely grated

small handful of coriander, to serve

Method

STEP 1

Toss the courgettes and sweet potatoes in 1 tsp olive oil, then tip onto a baking sheet lined with baking paper and bake at 200C/180C fan/gas 6 for 25 mins until the vegetables are tender and slightly charred. Boil the kettle.

STEP 2

Tip the red onion slices into a heatproof bowl, cover with boiling water from the kettle, then drain. Return to the bowl and mix with the lime juice. Set aside until needed.

STEP 3

Heat the remaining oil in a frying pan over a medium heat. Add the onion and thyme, cover and cook for 5-10 mins until the onion has started to soften. Tip in the tomatoes and a can of water, then add the bouillon powder, peanut butter, raisins, smoked paprika and chilli flakes, if using. Drop in the cinnamon stick, then cover and simmer for 20 mins.

STEP 4

Meanwhile, tip the black beans into a small pan with the liquid from the can, the cumin and garlic. Simmer over a low heat for 5-10 mins, then roughly mash with a fork.

STEP 5

Spoon half the sauce over two plates and top with half the roasted veg. Spoon over the beans and pickled red onions, then scatter with coriander before serving. Leftovers should be left to cool completely then keep chilled for up to two days. Reheat the sauce in a pan with a splash of water and microwave the beans and vegetables until piping hot.

Mediterranean fish gratins

Ingredients

3 tbsp olive oil

1 large onion, thinly sliced

1 fennel bulb (about 250g/9oz), trimmed and thinly sliced

3 large garlic cloves, finely sliced

1 heaped tsp coriander seeds, lightly crushed

150ml white wine

2 x 400g cans chopped tomatoes with herbs

2 tbsp tomato purée

good pinch of saffron

1 bay leaf

1 tbsp fresh lemon juice

1 small bunch flat-leaf parsley, leaves roughly chopped

900g mixed skinless fish fillets, (anything you like) cut into chunks

350g raw peeled king prawn

75g finely grated parmesan

50g panko or coarse dried breadcrumbs

green salad, to serve (optional)

Method

STEP 1

Heat the oil in a large, wide non-stick saucepan or sauté pan and gently fry the onion, fennel, garlic and coriander seeds for 15 mins, stirring regularly until the vegetables are softened and lightly coloured. Pour the wine into the pan and add the tomatoes, tomato purée, saffron and bay leaf. Season and bring to a gentle simmer. Cook for about 15 mins, stirring occasionally, until thick.

STEP 2

Heat oven to 220C/200C fan/gas 7. Stir the lemon juice and most of the parsley into the tomato mixture, pop the raw fish pieces and prawns on top and stir well. Cover tightly with a lid and simmer gently over a medium heat for 4-5 mins or until the fish is almost cooked. Stir a couple of times as the fish cooks, taking care not to let it break up.

STEP 3

Ladle the hot tomato and fish mixture into 6 individual pie dishes – they will each need to hold around 350ml. Mix the cheese, breadcrumbs, remaining parsley and a little ground black pepper together and sprinkle over the top. Bake on a baking tray for 20 mins or until the pies are golden brown and bubbling. Serve with green salad, if you like.

Cauliflower, paneer & pea curry

Ingredients

2 tbsp sunflower oil

225g pack paneer, cut into cubes

1 head of cauliflower broken into small florets

2 onions, thickly sliced

2 garlic cloves, crushed

2 heaped tbsp tikka masala paste

500g carton passata

200g frozen peas

small pack coriander, roughly chopped

basmati rice or naan breads, to serve

raita or your favourite chutney, to serve

Method

STEP 1

Heat 1 tbsp of oil in a large non-stick frying pan, add the paneer and fry gently until crisp. Remove with a slotted spoon and set aside. Add the remaining oil and the cauliflower to the pan, and cook for 10 mins until browned. Add the onions, and a little more oil if needed, and cook for a further 5 mins until softened. Stir in the garlic and curry paste, then pour in the passata and 250ml water, and season. Bring to a simmer, then cover and cook for 18-20 mins or until the cauliflower is just tender.

STEP 2

Add the frozen peas and crispy paneer to the pan and cook for a further 5 mins. Stir through most of the coriander and garnish with the rest. Serve with basmati rice or naan bread, raita or your favourite chutney.

Soy-baked potatoes with tuna sriracha mayo

Ingredients

4 large baking potatoes

3 x 135g cans tuna chunks in brine, drained

2 tbsp mayonnaise

2 ½ tbsp natural yogurt

4 spring onions, thinly sliced

1 thumb-sized piece of ginger, peeled and finely grated

1 lemon, juiced

2 tsp sriracha or hot sauce

3 pickled gherkins, finely chopped (optional)

2 tbsp reduced-salt soy sauce

320g spinach

For the dressing

1 tbsp extra virgin olive oil

2 tbsp cider vinegar

¼ tsp wholegrain mustard

Method

STEP 1

Prick the potatoes all over using a fork, then microwave on high for 10-15 mins, or until softened. Heat the oven to 200C/180C fan/gas 6, or turn on the air-fryer.

STEP 2

Tip the tuna into a bowl and mix with the mayo, yogurt, spring onions, ginger, half the lemon juice, the hot sauce and gherkins, if using.

STEP 3

When the potatoes are tender, score them lightly with a sharp knife, then pour over the soy sauce and toss quickly to coat. Bake in the oven for 15-20 mins or the air-fryer at 200C for 5 mins to crisp up the skins. Meanwhile, combine the dressing **Ingredients** with the remaining lemon juice and drizzle this over the spinach.

Split the potatoes in half, fill with the tuna mayo and serve with the spinach.

Healthy bolognese

Ingredients

100g wholewheat linguine

2 tsp rapeseed oil

1 fennel bulb, finely chopped

2 garlic cloves, sliced

200g pork mince with less than 5% fat

200g whole cherry tomatoes

1 tbsp balsamic vinegar

1 tsp vegetable bouillon powder

generous handful chopped basil

Method

STEP 1

Bring a large pan of water to the boil, then cook the linguine following pack instructions, about 10 mins.

STEP 2

Meanwhile, heat the oil in a non-stick wok or wide pan. Add the fennel and garlic and cook, stirring every now and then, until tender, about 10 mins.

STEP 3

Tip in the pork and stir-fry until it changes colour, breaking it up as you go so there are no large clumps. Add the tomatoes, vinegar and bouillon, then cover the pan and cook for 10 mins over a low heat until the tomatoes burst and the pork is cooked and tender. Add the linguine and basil and plenty of pepper, and toss well before serving.

STARTER RECIPES FOR VOLUME EATING

Sweetcorn chowder

Ingredients

1 tbsp sunflower oil

1 small onion, chopped

8 spring onions, sliced

400g new potatoes, peeled and halved

1l vegetable stock

500g sweetcorn kernels

200ml milk

small bunch of chives, chopped

Method

STEP 1

Heat the oil in a saucepan over a medium heat. Tip in the small chopped onions and most of the sliced spring onions (reserving around 2 tbsp) and fry for 6-8 mins, until soft but not golden. Scatter in the potatoes and fry for 4 mins, to soften a little, then pour in the stock and bring to a boil. Reduce the heat to medium-low and simmer for 15 mins. Season to taste, then tip in the sweetcorn and pour in the milk. Cook for 3-4 mins until the corn is tender. At this point, you can serve it chunky or blitz using a hand blender to break it up a little. Divide between bowls, then scatter over the chives before serving.

Beetroot carpaccio

Ingredients

3 beetroot, scrubbed

1 lemon, zested and juiced

2 tbsp olive oil

1 tbsp cider vinegar

2 tsp honey

1 tsp Dijon mustard

large handful of rocket

50g goat's cheese (optional)

20g walnuts, roughly chopped

Method

STEP 1

Trim away the ends of the beetroot then, using a mandoline or sharp knife, thinly slice into discs. Tip into a bowl and drizzle over half the lemon juice, half the olive oil and 1 tsp of the cider vinegar, then season well. Toss or mix together, cover with a clean tea towel and leave to marinate for 20 mins-1 hr.

STEP 2

Make a dressing by combining the remaining lemon juice, olive oil, cider vinegar, honey and the Dijon mustard with a good pinch of salt and freshly ground black pepper.

STEP 3

Arrange the beetroot slices on a platter, slightly overlapped in a spiral pattern, then pile the rocket into the middle, leaving most of the beetroot on display. Drizzle over the dressing, crumble over the goat's cheese, if using, and scatter with the chopped walnuts and lemon zest

Quick mushroom noodle soup

Ingredients

1 tsp sesame oil

75-100g mixed mushrooms

1 garlic clove, sliced

pinch of chilli flakes

400ml fresh vegetable or chicken stock or ½ stock cube

100g-150g ready-to-eat udon noodles

½ pak choi

large splash of soy sauce

squeeze of lime juice

1 tsp crispy chilli in oil

Method

STEP 1

Heat the sesame oil in a large, deep saucepan over a medium heat and fry the mushrooms for 3-4 mins until evenly coloured. Add the garlic and chilli flakes, and cook for another minute.

STEP 2

Add the stock (or crumble in the stock cube and add 400ml water), and bring to the boil. Tip in the noodles and pak choi, reduce the heat and simmer for 3-4 mins until the noodles are warmed through. Ladle the soup into a bowl and season with a splash of soy sauce, squeeze of lime juice and the crispy chilli in oil. Serve straightaway.

Vegan leek & potato soup

Ingredients

1 tbsp rapeseed oil, plus a drizzle to serve (optional)

2 large garlic cloves, chopped

500g leeks, thinly sliced

500g potatoes, cut into cubes

500ml vegan vegetable stock, made with 1½ tsp bouillon powder

500ml unsweetened almond milk

chopped chives and bread, to serve

Method

STEP 1

Heat the oil in a large pan over a medium heat and fry the garlic and leeks, stirring, until the veg has started to soften. Add the potatoes and stock, then cover and simmer for 15 mins until the leeks and potatoes are soft.

STEP 2

Pour in the almond milk, then remove from the heat and blitz using a hand blender until almost smooth, with a slightly chunky texture. Or, if you prefer, blitz until completely smooth. Reheat over a low heat if needed, then ladle into bowls and scatter with chives, drizzle with a little oil and serve with bread, if you like. Can be frozen for up to three months.

Black bean & tortilla soup

Ingredients

2 tbsp olive oil

1 chopped onion

2 chopped peppers

3 crushed garlic cloves

2 tsp ground cumin

1 tsp garlic granules

1 tsp chilli powder

2 tbsp tomato purée

1l veg stock

400g can chopped tomatoes

2 tbsp cornmeal or polenta

2 tbsp chopped pickled jalapeños

2 x 400g cans black beans

jalapeño brine

4 small corn tortillas

chopped coriander, avocado, crumbled feta and pumpkin seeds, to serve, if you like

Method

STEP 1

Heat the olive oil in a deep pan over a medium heat. Add the onion, peppers (any colour you like) and garlic cloves with a big pinch of salt. Cook for 10 mins, until starting to soften, then add the ground cumin, garlic granules and chilli powder along with the tomato purée. Cook for 5 mins, until the purée has caramelised.

STEP 2

Pour in the veg stock, chopped tomatoes, cornmeal or polenta, chopped pickled jalapeños and black beans, along with the liquid. Add a splash of jalapeño brine and bring to a simmer. Cook for 45 mins, until thickened and reduced. Season, then scatter in the corn tortillas, cut into small strips. (Use flour tortillas if that's what you have.) Rest for 5 mins before serving. Serve with chopped coriander, avocado, crumbled feta and pumpkin seeds, if you like.

Chunky peanut soup

Ingredients

2tbsp rapeseed oil

onions, chopped (320g)

1tbsp chopped ginger

3 large garlic cloves, chopped

1 fresh chilli, deseeded and chopped

2tbsp mild curry powder

1tsp cumin seeds

400g can chopped tomatoes

1.2l boiling vegetable stock, made with 3 tsp vegetable
bouillon

3tbsp chunky peanut butter

2tbsp tomato purée

400g potatoes, unpeeled and diced

320g butternut squash, finely diced

400g can chickpeas, drained

200g Savoy cabbage, shredded

⅓ x 30g pack fresh coriander, chopped

Method

STEP 1

Heat the oil in a large pan (it makes a big quantity) and fry the onions and ginger, stirring frequently, for 10 mins until starting to turn golden. Add the garlic and chilli, cook for a few mins more, then stir in the curry powder and cumin seeds.

STEP 2

Pour in the tomatoes and stock, add the peanut butter and tomato purée, then bring to the boil. Stir in the potatoes, squash, chickpeas and cabbage, then cover the pan and leave to simmer for 15 mins until the vegetables are tender. Stir in the fresh coriander, then spoon two portions into two bowls and serve. Cool and chill the remainder to eat another day. Will keep chilled for up to three days. To serve, reheat in a pan until piping hot.

Miso lentil & cabbage soup

Ingredients

1 tbsp olive oil

150g pancetta or chopped bacon

300g sliced mushrooms

1 tbsp olive oil

1 chopped onion

4 chopped garlic cloves

4 unpeeled sliced carrots

3 sliced sticks of celery

2 tbsp miso

500ml vegetable stock

200g washed and drained dried green lentils

½ head of chopped white cabbage

spoonful of thick yogurt

Method

STEP 1

Heat the olive oil in a deep pan over a medium-high heat. You can make this completely veggie, but if you have around 150g pancetta or chopped bacon to use, tip this in and brown all over before removing with a slotted spoon. Stir in the sliced mushrooms and brown all over before transferring to a bowl.

STEP 2

Pour in the olive oil, then tip in the chopped onion, the garlic cloves, sliced carrots and sticks of celery, leaves and all. Cook gently for 10 mins, until lightly softened. Stir in the miso, preferably red or brown, vegetable stock and 1 litre water and bring to a simmer.

STEP 3

Finally, stir in the washed and drained dried green lentils and head of chopped white cabbage. Tip the bacon and mushrooms back in. Cover and simmer gently for 30-35 mins until the lentils are tender. Season well and serve with a spoonful of thick yogurt.

Potato soup

Ingredients

1½ litres vegetable or chicken stock

5 potatoes, peeled and diced

1 carrot, peeled and diced

2 bay leaves

5 allspice berries

1 tbsp butter

1 onion, diced

1 tbsp plain flour

2 tbsp vegetable oil

2 slices of bread, cut into cubes

1 parsley, chopped

Optional topping

50g sausage, sliced and fried

Method

STEP 1

Put the stock in a large pan and bring to a simmer, then add the potatoes and carrots along with the bay leaves and allspice berries. Cover with a lid and cook over a medium-low heat for 30 mins, or until the vegetables are very tender.

STEP 2

Heat the butter in a frying pan and fry the onion for 8-10 mins or until soft and lightly golden. Add the flour, stir to make a paste (or roux) and cook until golden. Add 2 tbsp of the stock from the veg to the roux and stir until smooth, then scrape this into the rest of the stock and stir until combined. Bring the mixture back to a simmer and cook for 1 hr. The potatoes will break down and the soup will thicken.

STEP 3

Heat the oil in a frying pan and fry the bread until browned and crisp. Season well, then scatter across the soup with the chopped parsley. You can also add slices of fried sausage to the soup, if you like.

Cheesy cauliflower flask soup

Ingredients

1 cauliflower (about 1kg)

1 tbsp olive oil

1 onion, finely chopped

2 celery sticks, finely chopped

1 garlic clove, crushed

small handful of thyme

1 large potato (about 340g), cut into chunks

500ml milk

600ml vegetable stock

100g mature cheddar, grated

For the croutons

200g sourdough or other crusty bread, torn into bite-sized chunks

1 tsp dried mixed herbs

1 tsp garlic granules

25g parmesan or vegetarian alternative, finely grated

2 tbsp olive oil

Method

STEP 1

Trim the cauliflower and discard any wilted leaves, then roughly chop the florets, stalk and remaining leaves.

Heat the oil in a large, deep saucepan over a medium heat, tip in all the cauliflower pieces, the onion, celery, garlic, thyme and a large pinch of salt, cover partially with a lid and cook for 15-20 mins until all the vegetables have softened.

STEP 2

Tip in the potatoes, milk and stock, and bring to a simmer. Season well with black pepper, then continue to simmer for 15-20 mins, partially covered, until everything is fall-apart tender. Remove from the heat and discard the thyme. Blitz until smooth using a hand blender, then return to a low heat and stir in the cheese until fully melted. Season and add a splash more stock or milk if it's too thick. Will keep chilled for up to three days, or frozen for two months. If travelling, decant into a heatproof flask.

STEP 3

To make the croutons, heat the oven to 190C/170C fan/gas 5. Tip all the **Ingredients** onto a large baking tray and toss together using your hands. Season and bake for 15-17 mins until golden. Leave to cool completely on the tray. Will keep in an airtight container for up to three days. Sprinkle a handful of croutons over the soup or into the flask just before serving.

Slow-cooker pumpkin soup

Ingredients

2 tbsp rapeseed oil

3 onions (480g), chopped

30g ginger, peeled and chopped

3 large garlic cloves, chopped

1½-2 tbsp medium curry powder

1 tsp ground coriander

½ tsp crushed dried chillies (optional)

1kg pumpkin or butternut squash (flesh only), cut into cubes

1 tbsp vegetable bouillon powder (ensure vegan, if needed)

400g can coconut milk

180g dried red lentils

15g coriander, chopped

Method

STEP 1

Heat the oil in a large pan over a medium heat and fry the onions and ginger for 10 mins, stirring occasionally until softened and starting to colour. Stir in the garlic, curry powder, ground coriander and dried chillies, if using, and cook for 1 min more.

STEP 2

Tip the mixture into a large slow cooker along with all the remaining ingredients, except the fresh coriander. Add 2 litres water. Cook for 8 hrs on high, or overnight for 15 hrs on low. Stir well, then blitz using a hand blender until smooth. Ladle into bowls and scatter over the fresh coriander to serve. Once completely cool, the soup will keep chilled in an airtight container for 48 hrs or frozen for up to two months. Reheat in a pan over a low heat or in the microwave until piping hot.

Cauliflower & broccoli soup with seedy crumble

Ingredients

1 cauliflower (about 700g)

1 broccoli (about 450g)

2 tbsp vegetable or other flavourless oil

1 large onion, finely chopped

2 celery sticks, finely chopped

2 carrots, finely chopped

3 large garlic cloves, finely chopped

2 tsp ground cumin

1 tsp ground coriander

1 litre vegetable stock

For the crumble

2 tsp vegetable or other flavourless oil

50g fresh or dried breadcrumbs

25g mixed seeds

pinch of chilli flakes

25g parmesan or vegetarian alternative, finely grated

Method

STEP 1

Remove any wilted or brown leaves from the cauliflower. Cut the cauliflower and broccoli into bite-size florets, then finely chop the stalks and remaining leaves. Heat the oil in a large, deep saucepan over a medium heat and cook all the stalks and leaves, the onion, celery, carrot and garlic, partially covered with a lid, for 10 mins until everything is slightly softened. Remove the lid and stir in the spices and stock. Bring to a simmer, cook for 5 mins, then stir in the cauliflower and broccoli florets. Continue cooking, covered, for 10 mins more until everything is tender. Remove from the heat and blitz using a hand blender until thick and creamy. Season to taste.

STEP 2

Meanwhile, for the crumble, heat the oil in a small pan over a medium heat and toast the breadcrumbs, seeds and chilli flakes for 4-5 mins until golden and fragrant. Remove from the heat, season and stir in the cheese. Sprinkle the crumble over the soup to serve.

SIDE DISH RECIPES FOR VOLUME EATING

Chickpea salad

Ingredients

400g can chickpeas, drained and rinsed

small pack coriander, roughly chopped

small pack parsley, roughly chopped

1 red onion, thinly sliced

2 large tomatoes, chopped

2 tbsp olive oil

2 tbsp harissa

1 lemon, juiced

Method

STEP 1

Mix all the **Ingredients** together, mashing a little so the chickpeas are a bit rough round the edges – this helps absorb the dressing. (Can be made a day ahead and kept in the fridge.) Try it with slow-cooked Greek lamb and tzatziki sauce.

Cauliflower rice

Ingredients

1 medium cauliflower

good handful coriander, chopped

cumin seeds, toasted (optional)

Our Most Popular Alternative

Spicy cauliflower & halloumi rice

Method

STEP 1

Cut the hard core and stalks from the cauliflower and pulse the rest in a food processor to make grains the size of rice. Tip into a heatproof bowl, cover with cling film, then pierce and microwave for 7 mins on high – there is no need to add any water. Stir in the coriander. For spicier rice, add some toasted cumin seeds.

Roasted aubergine salad

Ingredients

2 aubergines, chopped

2 red peppers, chopped

2 small red onions, peeled and cut into 8 wedges

6 garlic cloves, skin left on

6 tbsp olive oil

200g cherry tomatoes

400g can chickpeas, drained and rinsed

3 tbsp pomegranate molasses

1 lemon, juiced

½ tsp honey

2 tbsp capers

60g rocket leaves

4 tbsp sunflower or pumpkin seeds

Method

STEP 1

Heat the oven to 200C/180C fan/gas 6. Scatter the aubergines, peppers, onion wedges and garlic cloves into a large roasting tin, season with salt and pepper, then drizzle over 4 tbsp olive oil. Mix well using your hands to ensure everything is coated in the oil. Put in the oven for 30 mins, then remove and tip in the cherry tomatoes and chickpeas. Mix to combine and put back in the oven for 20 mins until everything is roasted. Remove from the oven and set aside to cool.

STEP 2

Meanwhile, make the dressing by combining 2 tbsp of the pomegranate molasses with the lemon juice, honey, capers, remaining oil and a good pinch of salt and pepper. Tip the cooled aubergine mix into a serving bowl with the rocket and dressing, then gently toss to combine everything. Scatter over the sunflower or pumpkin seeds and drizzle over the remaining pomegranate molasses.

Spring green fattoush

Ingredients

500g broad beans, frozen or fresh

1 cucumber

3 wholemeal pitta breads

zest and juice 1 lemon

4 tbsp olive oil

1 tsp caster sugar

20g bunch mint, smaller leaves picked, rest very roughly chopped

20g bunch flat-leaf parsley, very roughly chopped

small bunch chives, snipped

170g feta cheese, crumbled

1 tbsp white wine vinegar

1 tsp honey

¼ small bunch of chives, roughly chopped

1 tsp Dijon mustard

Method

STEP 1

First make the dressing. Whisk the **Ingredients** together with a good pinch each of salt and freshly ground black pepper, or shake together in a jar until emulsified.

STEP 2

Trim the courgettes, then cut into long ribbons using a vegetable peeler. Tip into a large bowl with the tomatoes, beans, salad leaves and herbs, and toss everything together using your hands to combine.

STEP 3

Drizzle over the dressing and scatter over the parmesan shavings, toss again and tip into a salad bowl or platter to serve.

Tuna, asparagus & white bean salad

Ingredients

1 large bunch asparagus

2 x cans tuna steaks in water, drained

2 x cans cannellini beans in water, drained

1 red onion, very finely chopped

2 tbsp capers

1 tbsp olive oil

1 tbsp red wine vinegar

2 tbsp tarragon, finely chopped

Method

STEP 1

Cook the asparagus in a large pan of boiling water for 4-5 mins until tender. Drain well, cool under running water, then cut into finger-length pieces. Toss together the tuna, beans, onion, capers and asparagus in a large serving bowl.

STEP 2

Mix the oil, vinegar and tarragon together, then pour over the salad. Chill until ready to serve.

Deconstructed guacamole

Ingredients

2 tomatoes, finely chopped

4 tsp finely chopped red onion

2 tsp finely chopped coriander

1 small avocado, halved and stoned

pinch of chilli powder, hot or mild, to taste

2 small lime wedges, to serve

Method

STEP 1

Mix the tomatoes, onion and coriander in a bowl. Spoon onto the avocado halves, sprinkle with a little chilli powder, then serve with a lime wedge each for squeezing over.

Sea bass with sizzled ginger, chilli & spring onions

Ingredients

Take off the heat and toss in the bunch of shredded spring onions. Splash the fish with 1 tbsp soy sauce and spoon over the contents of the pan.

Chicken chop suey

Ingredients

2 tbsp vegetable oil

1 large chicken breast, cut into thin bite-sized slices

1 onion, sliced

2 garlic cloves, roughly chopped or minced

1 carrot, sliced

½ tbsp dark soy sauce

½ tsp chicken powder or a pinch of salt

½ tsp sugar

pinch of white pepper (essential as it totally changes the flavour of the dish)

2 spring onions, chopped into slivers

100g ready-to-eat beansprouts

1 tbsp cornflour, mixed with 2 tbsp water

1 tsp sesame oil

steamed white rice or fried noodles, to serve

Method

STEP 1

Heat a wok over a high heat and, once hot, pour in the oil. Add the chicken and fan out in a single layer so that it's in direct contact with the hot wok. Once it has started to brown on one side, give it a good stir, then toss in the onion and garlic. Stir, then add the carrots, dark soy, chicken powder or salt, sugar, white pepper and spring onions. Stir, then add the beansprouts and fry, stirring, for 1 min before pouring in 50ml just-boiled water.

STEP 2

Bring to the boil, then slowly pour in the cornflour paste to loosen it, mixing at the same time to prevent any lumps. Once the sauce has thickened, switch off the heat and add the sesame oil. Serve on a bed of steamed white rice or freshly fried noodles.

PART V: INCORPORATING HEALTHY VOLUME EATING HABITS

C onsciously incorporating nutrient-dense, portion-controlled, and health-promoting food selections into one's diet is the cornerstone of good volume eating habits. Eating more whole, unprocessed foods that are high in hydration, fiber, and minerals is one way to improve your health. For example, fruits and vegetables are great options for healthy volume eating since they are dense in nutrients and have minimal calories per serving.

Including a variety of foods that are rich in different macronutrients and micronutrients is essential for a

vegetables high in water content, such watermelon and cucumbers, can help keep you hydrated all day long.

A healthy volume eating plan should include a variety of meals that are rich in nutrients, a good attitude toward food, conscious portion management, and a focus on nutritional density. A person's quest for health and wellbeing may be advanced by adopting these practices, which provide a gratifying and long-term strategy for food consumption.

Lifestyle Adjustments

In order to live a better and more balanced existence, it is essential to make changes to one's lifestyle. Diet, exercise, stress management, and sleep habits are just a few areas that frequently undergo these kinds of transformations. Making better food choices, practicing mindful eating, and controlling portions are all part of a more attentive approach to nutrition, which is a big change in lifestyle. Weight loss, increased energy, and general health can all result from this in the long run.

Getting regular exercise is another important part of making changes to your lifestyle. Heart health, muscular strength, and mental well-being are all improved when exercise is a regular part of people's lives, whether it's through organized exercises or more casual pursuits like walking or cycling. A more active lifestyle and a better attitude towards fitness can be achieved by engaging in activities that provide joy and satisfaction.

Managing stress effectively is essential for general well-being. To that end, one way to modify one's way of life is to make time each day to practice relaxation techniques like deep breathing, meditation, or mindfulness. One way to improve one's mental health and ability to deal with life's difficulties is to make time for things that make one happy and relaxed.

An essential part of maintaining a healthy lifestyle is getting enough good sleep. Improve your sleep quality by making some changes to your daily routine, such as sticking to a regular sleep schedule, making your bedroom a relaxing place to sleep, and developing rituals to help you wind down at the end of the day. Cognitive performance, emotional stability, and physical health are all positively impacted by getting a good night's sleep.

The key to a happy life is having good friends and a community that has your back. Making changes to one's way of life in this area may entail engaging in more social activities, reaching out for help when you need it, and fostering and maintaining connections. Having supportive friends and family may help you weather tough times, make you feel like you belong, and boost your happiness levels.

A second essential change is striking a balance between one's professional and personal life. Improve your work-life balance by learning to say "no," making self-care a priority, and learning to manage your time wisely. A more sustainable and satisfying way of life may be achieved by valuing leisure time and doing things you like.

Making changes to one's way of life may have a positive impact on one's health in all areas of life. A better and more satisfying life may be yours with little to no effort put into your food, level of physical exercise, stress management, quality of sleep, social networks, or work-life balance. People may build a lifestyle that promotes their health and happiness in the long run by making little, manageable adjustments.

PART VI: VOLUME EATING AND YOUR JOURNEY TO A BETTER YOU

Foods that are both high in nutritious content and low in calories is central to the volume eating philosophy, which provides a long-term, comprehensive strategy for improving one's diet. We have now covered the basics of volume eating, its concepts and tenets, and how it affects satiety, weight control, and general health.

Fruits, vegetables, whole grains, lean meats, and other nutrient-dense foods with little calories are highlighted. Not only can these options help you feel full longer, but they also supply your body with nutrients it needs, including vitamins, minerals, and antioxidants. A well-rounded approach to meeting nutritional demands may be achieved by adding high-volume meals in the diet, which help maintain a balanced intake of macronutrients including fiber, carbs, proteins, and healthy fats.

Critical components of volume eating, which promote a healthy connection with food and minimize overconsumption, are portion management and mindful eating. People can eat more without sacrificing their calorie objectives if they pay attention to signals that tell them when they are full or hungry. To help achieve fullness while controlling calorie consumption, try starting your meal plan with low-calorie, high-volume components.

Changes to one's way of life outside one's food choices are essential for the long-term success of volume eating. An all-encompassing and satisfying lifestyle includes balancing other nutrients, engaging in regular physical activity, controlling stress, prioritizing sleep, and cultivating social ties. Along with the concepts of volume eating, these modifications help create a balanced approach to health.

A practical and adaptable attitude, one that permits occasional treats and acknowledges that eating patterns may fluctuate, is necessary to sustain a volume eating regimen. For this strategy to work in the long run, you need to be consistent about drinking enough of water, eating a variety of foods, and making well-informed dietary choices. Adopting these habits can help individuals have a healthy relationship with food, which in turn promotes their physical and mental health and helps them lead a more fulfilling life.

Maintaining the Volume Eating Diet

Keeping to a volume eating plan requires developing habits that last and making decisions that benefit your health in the long run. Maintaining a focus on low-calorie, nutrient-dense meals is an important tactic. Eating a diet rich in fruits, vegetables, whole grains, and lean meats on a regular basis is a great way to acquire all the nutrients you need without going overboard on calories. In addition to aiding with weight loss, this method improves general health by supplying the body with antioxidants, minerals, and vitamins.

Maintaining a volume eating regimen requires consistent portion management. Some helpful strategies to help you maintain a healthy relationship with food include learning to recognize when you're full, utilizing smaller dishes, and avoiding mindless eating. One way to keep from going overboard on calories while yet enjoying the advantages of larger servings is to be conscious of portion proportions.

For a volume eating diet to be successful in the long run, one must be willing to be flexible and have a realistic outlook. Maintaining a healthy diet is easier when you give yourself permission to indulge every once in a while and accept that eating habits could change depending on the situation. Instead of imposing rigid standards, we should encourage healthy eating habits that work for people and help them develop a positive connection with food.

The maintenance of a volume eating diet also requires continuing to vary meal selections. One way to keep meals interesting and promote nutritional satisfaction is to try new dishes, try various fruits and vegetables, and add diverse flavors and textures. The diet becomes more maintainable with time because of the diversity that guarantees a broad spectrum of nutrients and helps prevent boredom.

A volume eating diet relies heavily on meal preparation and planning. To reduce consumption of unhealthy convenience foods, it is helpful to plan meals ahead of time, keep healthy snacks on hand, and make nutritious meals at home. Maintaining adherence to the selected eating pattern is made easier by cultivating an atmosphere that encourages the volume eating method.

One of the most basic rules of a volume eating regimen is to drink enough of water. If you want to feel full on fewer calories and avoid overeating, drink water often throughout the day, but particularly before meals. Fruits and vegetables are high in water, so eating them might help you stay hydrated and full for longer.

Finally, choosing nutrient-dense foods consistently, controlling portions, having a flexible mentality, eating a variety of foods, and planning meals effectively are all sustainable behaviors that are necessary to maintain a volume eating diet. Individuals may reap the long-term advantages of a volume eating strategy, which promote physical and mental well-being, by integrating these practices into their everyday lives.

Printed in Great Britain
by Amazon